LOW POTASSIUM COOKBOOK

MAIN COURSE – 80 + Quick and easy to prepare at home recipes, step-by-step low potassium recipes to improve kidney disease and avoid dialysis

TABLE OF CONTENTS

BREAKFAST 7

CHEESE AND GARLIC WEDGES 7

PARMESAN CRAKCKERS 9

SESAME TWIST 10

OAT BISCUITS 11

TOFU SCRAMBLE WITH POTATOES 12

OVERNIGHT OATS 13

AVOCADO TOAST 14

GOAT CHEESE AND PARSLEY SCRAMBLE 15

VANILLA PUDDING 16

BANANA PANCAKES 17

COCONUT QUINOA 18

TOMATO SCRAMBLE 19

BREAKFAST BURRITO 20

PINEAPPLE PUDDING 21

SRIRACHA BREAKFAST BOWL 22

VEGAN PANCAKES 23

BROWNBAG BURRITOS 24

OAT PANCAKES 25

BANANA BRUSCHETTA 26

FRENCH TOAST 27

LUNCH 28

CHICKEN SOUP 28

CAULIFLOWER SOUP 30

CHICKEN STEW WITH MUSHROOMS 32

CHILI THAI SAUCE 34

GRILLED BEAK STEAK 36

PANINI 38

TOFU STIR-FRY 39

SESAME ASPARAGUS 41

BASIL PESTO WITH PASTA 42

COUSCOUS SALAD 43

TOFU STICKS 45

BAKED EGGPLANT FRIES 46

PITA CHIPS 48

ROASTED RED PEPPER DIP 49

CHICKEN IN MUSHROOM SAUCE 50

BARBECUE CHICKEN SALAD 52

TUNA SPREAD 54

THAI SALAD 55

PARSLEY PILAF 57

STEAMED FISH 58

SHRIMP STIR FRY 60

DINNER 62

LOW POTASSIUM FRIED POTATOES 62

STEWED POTATOES 63

LOW POTASSIUM STIR-FRY 65

LOW POTASSIUM SOY SAUCE 67

GUACAMOLE 68

GREEN PEA CASSEROLE 69

TUNA CASSEROLE 71

PASTA SALAD	72
LINGUINE	73
SPAGHETTI WITH GARLIC	74
PIZZA	75
RICE WITH HERBES	77
BUFFALO CHICKEN DIP	78
SAUTEED APPLES	79
CELERY STUFFING	80
STUFFED JALAPENOS	81
FRIED CABBAGE	82
ZUCCHINI BREAD	83
PINWHEELS	85
RICE PILAF	87
SNACKS & DRINKS	**88**
RASPBERRY PEAR SORBET	88
RASPBERRY LIMEADE	90
GRILLED CORN	91
CANDY GRAPES	92
GINGER COOKIES	93
PUMPKIN PIE	95
APPLE CAKE	96
CHOCOLATE CAKE	98
BLUEBERRY SMOOTHIE	99
PINEAPPLE SMOOTHIE	100
FRUITS SMOOTHIE	101
MIXED BERRY SMOOTHIE	102

PEACH SMOOTHIE	103
STRAWBERRY SMOOTHIE	104
BANANA SMOOTHIE	105
APPLE SMOOTHIE	106
EGG SHAKE	107
MANGO SMOOTHIE	108

☞Copyright 2018 by Noah Jerris - All rights reserved.

This document is geared towards providing exact and reliable information in regards to the topic and issue covered. The publication is sold with the idea that the publisher is not required to render accounting, officially permitted, or otherwise, qualified services. If advice is necessary, legal or professional, a practiced individual in the profession should be ordered.

- From a Declaration of Principles which was accepted and approved equally by a Committee of the American Bar Association and a Committee of Publishers and Associations.

In no way is it legal to reproduce, duplicate, or transmit any part of this document in either electronic means or in printed format. Recording of this publication is strictly prohibited and any storage of this document is not allowed unless with written permission from the publisher. All rights reserved.

The information provided herein is stated to be truthful and consistent, in that any liability, in terms of inattention or otherwise, by any usage or abuse of any policies, processes, or directions contained within is the solitary and utter responsibility of the recipient reader. Under no circumstances will any legal responsibility or blame be held against the publisher for any reparation, damages, or monetary loss due to the information herein, either directly or indirectly.

Respective authors own all copyrights not held by the publisher.

The information herein is offered for informational purposes solely, and is universal as so. The presentation of the information is without contract or any type of guarantee assurance.

The trademarks that are used are without any consent, and the publication of the trademark is without permission or backing by the trademark owner. All trademarks and brands within this book are for clarifying purposes only and are the owned by the owners themselves, not affiliated with this document.

Introduction

Low potassium recipes for personal enjoyment but also for family enjoyment. You will love them for sure for how easy it is to prepare them.

BREAKFAST

CHEESE AND GARLIC WEDGES

Serves: **4**

Prep Time: **10** Minutes

Cook Time: **30** Minutes

Total Time: **40** Minutes

INGREDIENTS

- 3 pita bread
- ¼ lb. low-salt margarine
- 2 cloves garlic
- 2 tablespoons basil
- ½ cup parmesan cheese

DIRECTIONS

1. Preheat oven to 325 F
2. Split pita bread in half and cut into 4 wedges
3. Mix basil, garlic and margarine
4. Brush bread with mixture and sprinkle with parmesan cheese

5. Place in a single payer on oven and bake for 8-10 minutes or until crisp
6. Remove and serve

PARMESAN CRAKCKERS

Serves: **4**

Prep Time: **10** Minutes

Cook Time: **10** Minutes

Total Time: **20** Minutes

INGREDIENTS

- 6 tablespoons low-salt margarine
- 1 cup parmesan cheese
- 1 egg yolk
- ½ cup water
- 2 cups plain flour

DIRECTIONS

1. Preheat oven to 350 F
2. In a bowl mix flour with margarine, add egg yolk, cheese and mix well
3. Add water to the dough and divide dough into 2 portions
4. Cut into individual crackers and place on a baking sheet
5. Bake for 8-10 minutes or until brown, remove and serve

SESAME TWIST

Serves: **4**

Prep Time: **10** Minutes

Cook Time: **30** Minutes

Total Time: **40** Minutes

INGREDIENTS

- 2 oz. low salt margarine
- 2 tablespoons sesame seeds
- 2 tablespoons parmesan cheese
- 2 tablespoons poppy seeds

DIRECTIONS

1. Preheat oven to 350 F
2. Cut pastry sheets in half and brush with butter
3. Mix cheese, sesame seeds and poppy
4. Sprinkle over pastry and cut into small strips
5. Place into greased baking trays and bake for 8-10 minutes or until golden brown
6. Remove and serve

OAT BISCUITS

Serves: **4**

Prep Time: **10** Minutes

Cook Time: **30** Minutes

Total Time: **40** Minutes

INGREDIENTS

- ½ cup sugar
- 1/3 lb. low-salt margarine
- 1 tablespoon honey
- 1 cup flour
- 1 tsp baking powder
- ¼ tsp cinnamon
- 1 cup oats

DIRECTIONS

1. Preheat oven to 300 F
2. Cream margarine, honey and sugar, sift cinnamon, flour and baking powder
3. Add oats to the mixture and roll mixture into balls
4. Place on a greased oven tray and bake for 12-15 minutes or until golden brown, remove and serve

TOFU SCRAMBLE WITH POTATOES

Serves: **4**

Prep Time: **10** Minutes

Cook Time: **15** Minutes

Total Time: **25** Minutes

INGREDIENTS
- 5 oz. tofu
- 1 cup mushrooms
- 1 cup onions
- 1 sweet potato
- 1 tablespoon coconut oil
- 1 cup spinach

DIRECTIONS

1. **Wrap tofu in a towel and cover for a couple of minutes**
2. **Dice tofu and sweet potato**
3. **In a pan heat oil over medium heat and sauté tofu and potatoes**
4. **Add mushrooms, onions, spinach and sauté**
5. **Remove and serve**

OVERNIGHT OATS

Serves: 2
Prep Time: *10*   Minutes
Cook Time: *10*   Minutes
Total Time: *20*   Minutes

INGREDIENTS

- 1 tablespoon maple syrup
- 1 cup rolled oats
- 1 cup almond milk
- 1 tablespoon peanut butter
- 2 cup blueberries
- ¼ tablespoon cinnamon
- 1 banana
- 3 tablespoons chia seeds

DIRECTIONS

1. In a bowl mix all ingredients
2. Cover and refrigerate
3. Serve in the morning

AVOCADO TOAST

Serves: **2**

Prep Time: **10** Minutes

Cook Time: **10** Minutes

Total Time: **20** Minutes

INGREDIENTS

- 1 slice bread
- 1 tablespoon lemon juice
- ½ tsp pepper
- ½ avocado
- ½ tablespoon chia seeds
- 1/3 tablespoons sunflower seed

DIRECTIONS

1. Mash the avocado and combine with sunflower seeds and chia seeds
2. Add lemon juice, pepper and mix well
3. Spread onto the toast and top with seeds

GOAT CHEESE AND PARSLEY SCRAMBLE

Serves: 2
Prep Time: 10 Minutes
Cook Time: 10 Minutes
Total Time: 20 Minutes

INGREDIENTS

- 2 eggs
- ½ dash pepper
- 1 tsp olive oil
- ½ cup tomatoes
- 1 tablespoon parsley
- 1 oz. goat cheese
- 1 slice bread

DIRECTIONS

1. In a bowl whisk pepper and eggs
2. In a skillet heat oil and pour egg mixture and cook slowly
3. Add tomatoes and parsley and sprinkle with goat cheese
4. Cook for 1-2 minutes per side remove and serve

VANILLA PUDDING

Serves: **2**

Prep Time: **10** Minutes

Cook Time: **10** Minutes

Total Time: **20** Minutes

INGREDIENTS

- 1 cup almond milk
- 1 tablespoon maple syrup
- 1 tablespoon vanilla extract
- ¼ tsp cinnamon
- ¼ tsp ginger
- ½ tsp cardamom
- ½ tsp cloves
- 2 tablespoons chia seed

DIRECTIONS

1. In a container add all ingredients and whisk together until well incorporated
2. Refrigerate overnight, remove and serve

BANANA PANCAKES

Serves: **1**

Prep Time: **10** Minutes

Cook Time: **10** Minutes

Total Time: **20** Minutes

INGREDIENTS

- 1 egg
- 1 scoop protein powder
- 1 banana
- 1 stevia
- ½ tsp baking powder

DIRECTIONS

1. In a bowl mix all ingredients, mix until every ingredient is incorporated
2. Pour mixture into a skillet and cook for 1-2 minutes per side
3. Remove and serve

COCONUT QUINOA

Serves: **4**

Prep Time: **10** Minutes

Cook Time: **30** Minutes

Total Time: **40** Minutes

INGREDIENTS

- 1 cup quinoa
- 1 cup coconut milk
- 1 cup pumpkin and squash seeds
- 1 cup water
- 1 cup strawberries

DIRECTIONS

1. **In a pot add quinoa and coconut milk, stir in the rest of ingredients and boil**
2. **Lower the heat and simmer for 12-15 minutes**
3. **Add water if necessary**
4. **Divide into portions and top with berries**

TOMATO SCRAMBLE

Serves: **4**

Prep Time: **10** Minutes

Cook Time: **10** Minutes

Total Time: **20** Minutes

INGREDIENTS

- ½ tablespoon olive oil
- 2 tsp parsley
- 1 tsp pepper
- 1 slice bread
- 1 tomatoes
- 1 egg

DIRECTIONS

1. Chop tomato and fry with olive oil
2. Remove from pan and set aside
3. Scramble eggs, add tomatoes, parsley and pepper
4. Cook for 1-2 minutes per side, remove and serve

BREAKFAST BURRITO

Serves: **2**

Prep Time: **10** Minutes

Cook Time: **10** Minutes

Total Time: **20** Minutes

INGREDIENTS

- ½ cup brown rice
- 2 eggs
- 1 tablespoon salsa
- 1 tortilla
- 1 red bell pepper
- ½ avocado

DIRECTIONS

1. Chop bell pepper and avocado, set aside
2. In a bowl crack an egg and scramble, pour into a pan and cook on low heat
3. Combine egg with rice, bell pepper, salsa and avocado
4. Pour mixture into tortilla and serve

PINEAPPLE PUDDING

Serves: 2

Prep Time: 10 Minutes

Cook Time: 10 Minutes

Total Time: 20 Minutes

INGREDIENTS

- 1 cup almond milk
- 1 scoop protein powder
- ½ cup pineapple
- 1 tablespoon chia seeds

DIRECTIONS

1. In a container mix all ingredients
2. Refrigerate for at least one hour
3. Remove and serve

SRIRACHA BREAKFAST BOWL

Serves: **4**

Prep Time: **10** Minutes

Cook Time: **20** Minutes

Total Time: **30** Minutes

INGREDIENTS

- 1 cup rice
- 1 tsp soy sauce
- ¾ tsp sauce
- 6 tablespoons sesame oil
- ½ cup pineapple
- 1 stalk onion
- 1 egg
- 1 dash pepper

DIRECTIONS

1. **Cook rice according directions**
2. **Season with sriracha, sesame oil and soy sauce**
3. **Chop pineapple and slice onion and stir in rice**
4. **Fry the egg and season and top the rice bowl with the egg and serve**

VEGAN PANCAKES

Serves: **2**

Prep Time: **10** Minutes

Cook Time: **10** Minutes

Total Time: **20** Minutes

INGREDIENTS

- 1 cup almond milk
- 1 tsp nutmeg
- 1 tablespoon coconut oil
- 1 cup oats
- 1 banana
- ½ all purpose baking flour
- 2 tablespoons baking powder
- ½ tsp salt
- ½ tsp cinnamon

DIRECTIONS

1. In a blender blend oats and milk, add the rest of ingredients except coconut oil
2. In a pan heat coconut oil and pour pancake mixture
3. Cook for 2-3 minutes per side, remove and serve

BROWNBAG BURRITOS

Serves: **3**

Prep Time: **10** Minutes

Cook Time: **10** Minutes

Total Time: **20** Minutes

INGREDIENTS

- 2 tortilla
- 5 tablespoons cumin
- 1 can black beans
- 1 cup cheddar cheese
- 1 cup salsa
- 1 tablespoon chili powder

DIRECTIONS

1. In a pan add salsa, chili powder, cumin and beans
2. Cook over medium heat for 8-10 minutes
3. Spoon mixture into tortillas and top with cheese
4. Serve when ready

OAT PANCAKES

Serves: **2**

Prep Time: **10** Minutes

Cook Time: **10** Minutes

Total Time: **20** Minutes

INGREDIENTS

- 2/4 cup oats
- 2/4 cup almond milk
- 1 cup water
- 1 egg
- 1 tablespoon cinnamon
- ½ oz. coconut flour

DIRECTIONS

1. In a blender add oats, milk and water blend until smooth
2. Add an egg and stir
3. Add cinnamon, coconut flour and mix until well combine
4. Pour mixture into a pan and cook for 1-2 minutes per side, remove and serve

BANANA BRUSCHETTA

Serves: **2**

Prep Time: **10** Minutes

Cook Time: **10** Minutes

Total Time: **20** Minutes

INGREDIENTS

- 2 slices bread
- 1 tsp honey
- ½ oz. walnuts
- 2 oz. cottage cheese
- 2/3 cup banana
- ½ tsp cinnamon

DIRECTIONS

1. **Toast bread**
2. **Spread toast with cottage cheese and top with banana**
3. **Sprinkle with cinnamon, honey and walnuts**

FRENCH TOAST

Serves: *4*

Prep Time: *10* Minutes

Cook Time: *30* Minutes

Total Time: *40* Minutes

INGREDIENTS

- 2 slices bread
- 3 tablespoons butter
- 2 cup strawberries
- 1 cup milk
- 2 tablespoons sugar
- 2 egg

DIRECTIONS

1. Toast the bread
2. In a bowl mix sugar, eggs, milk and pour mixture over bread and refrigerate
3. Place slices of bread in a pan and sprinkle with sugar
4. Cook for 2-3 minutes, remove and serve

LUNCH

CHICKEN SOUP

Serves: **4**

Prep Time: **10** Minutes

Cook Time: **35** Minutes

Total Time: **45** Minutes

INGREDIENTS

- 2 cups Mirepoix
- 1 bay leaf
- 8 cups no salt chicken broth
- 2 boneless skinless chicken breast
- 1 cup baby carrot
- 1 cup baby carrot
- 1 tablespoon olive oil
- ¾ cup rice
- ¼ tsp pepper
- 3 thyme springs

DIRECTIONS

1. In a pot sauté carrot, onion, celery and olive oil

2. Add stock, bay leaf, rice, pepper and thyme and bring to boil
3. Reduce heat and simmer for 15-20 minutes
4. Add chicken and simmer for another 10-12 minutes
5. Remove bay leaf and serve

CAULIFLOWER SOUP

Serves: **4**

Prep Time: **10** Minutes

Cook Time: **60** Minutes

Total Time: **70** Minutes

INGREDIENTS

- 1 head cauliflower
- 1 clove garlic
- 1 tsp sage
- ½ tsp black pepper
- 5 cups chicken stock
- 1 head garlic
- 1 tsp olive oil
- 1 cup onion
- 1 cup apple
- 1 tsp thyme
- 1 tsp rosemary
- 8 baguette slices

DIRECTIONS

1. Preheat oven to 325 F
2. Drizzle garlic head with olive oil and wrap in aluminum foil and roast for 25-30 minutes
3. Place baguette slices on a baking sheet and toast for 10-12 minutes
4. Squeeze the softened garlic cloves on the baguette slices
5. In a sauce pan add vegetables, spices, chicken stock and bring to boil
6. Reduce heat ad simmer for 20-30 minutes
7. With a blender, puree soup and garnish with garlic
8. Serve with baguette slices

CHICKEN STEW WITH MUSHROOMS

Serves: *4*

Prep Time: *10* Minutes

Cook Time: *30* Minutes

Total Time: *40* Minutes

INGREDIENTS

- ½ cup onion
- 1 cup cooked chicken
- 1 cup no-salt chicken stock
- ¼ tablespoon seasoning
- ¼ tsp paprika
- ½ tsp garlic powder
- ¼ tsp black pepper
- 1 tablespoon cornstarch
- ¼ cup milk
- 1 clove garlic
- ¼ cup red pepper
- ¼ cup shitake mushrooms
- ¼ cup button mushrooms
- 1 cup kale
- 1 tablespoon olive oil

DIRECTIONS

1. Sauté the onions and garlic together in a skillet
2. Add onions and the rest of vegetables
3. Sauté until they are soft
4. Add chicken stock, spices, cooked chicken and dry spices
5. In another container mix milk and cornstarch
6. Add to stew and simmer
7. When ready serve with rice or noodles

CHILI THAI SAUCE

Serves: **4**

Prep Time: **10** Minutes

Cook Time: **10** Minutes

Total Time: **20** Minutes

INGREDIENTS

- 1 cup water
- 1 tsp pepper flakes
- 1 tsp ketchup
- 3 tsp cornstarch
- ¾ cup vinegar
- ¼ cup sugar
- 1 tsp ginger
- 1 tsp garlic
- 1 tsp garlic

DIRECTIONS

1. Boil water and vinegar
2. Add ginger, garlic, sugar, red pepper flakes and ketchup

3. Simmer for 5-10 minutes, add cornstarch and continue stirring, remove and serve

GRILLED BEAK STEAK

Serves: *4*

Prep Time: *10* Minutes

Cook Time: *20* Minutes

Total Time: *30* Minutes

INGREDIENTS

- 2 tablespoons olive oil
- 1 onion
- 1 baguette
- ½ bunch arugula
- 1 tablespoon wine vinegar
- 3 cloves garlic
- ½ tsp hot pepper flakes
- 1 lb. beef

DIRECTIONS

1. Mix vinegar, oil, garlic and pepper flakes in a bag and set aside
2. Add meat to marinade and refrigerate overnight
3. Remove steak from bag and grill steak for 4-5 minutes per side
4. Fry onion in a skillet and toss with marinade

5. Slice steak and top with onions and arugula

PANINI

Serves: **2**

Prep Time: **10** Minutes

Cook Time: **10** Minutes

Total Time: **20** Minutes

INGREDIENTS

- 3 Panini buns
- 1 cup egg plant
- 1 cup cooked roast beef
- 2 tablespoons mayonnaise
- 1 tablespoon pesto sauce

DIRECTIONS

1. Slice buns in half
2. In a bowl mix pesto sauce and mayonnaise and spread on each bun
3. Top with vegetables and roast beef

TOFU STIR-FRY

Serves: **4**

Prep Time: **10** Minutes

Cook Time: **10** Minutes

Total Time: **20** Minutes

INGREDIENTS

- 1 cup white rice
- 1 tablespoon hoisin sauce
- 1 tablespoon rice vinegar
- 1 tsp cornstarch
- 1 cloves garlic
- 1 jalapeno pepper
- ½ cup basil leaves
- 3 tablespoons canola oil
- 1 package tofu
- 1 eggplant
- 3 scallions

DIRECTIONS

1. **Cook rice following the package instructions**

2. In a skillet heat 1 tablespoon oil, add tofu and cook for 10-12 minutes
3. Transfer to a plate
4. Add vegetables and cook until tender, add sauce, toss and toss until thickened
5. Serve with basil and rice

SESAME ASPARAGUS

Serves: 2

Prep Time: 10 Minutes

Cook Time: 15 Minutes

Total Time: 25 Minutes

INGREDIENTS

- 12 asparagus
- 1 lemon juice
- 1 tablespoon sesame oil
- 1 tsp sesame seeds

DIRECTIONS

1. In a bowl mix lemon juice, sesame oil and sesame seeds
2. Wrap in tinfoil and bake at 350 for 15 minutes or until tender
3. Remove and serve

BASIL PESTO WITH PASTA

Serves: **2**

Prep Time: **10** Minutes

Cook Time: **20** Minutes

Total Time: **30** Minutes

INGREDIENTS

- 1/3 lb. pasta
- ½ cup Parmesan cheese
- ½ cup olive oil
- 1 cup basil
- 2 cloves garlic
- ½ cup pine nuts

DIRECTIONS

1. Cook pasta and set aside
2. In a bowl mix garlic, pine nuts and basil
3. Mix with Parmesan cheese and add oil
4. Serve over pasta

COUSCOUS SALAD

Serves: *1*

Prep Time: *10* Minutes

Cook Time: *10* Minutes

Total Time: *20* Minutes

INGREDIENTS

- 3 cup water
- ¼ tsp cumin
- 1 tablespoon honey
- 1 tsp lemon juice
- 1 green onion
- 1 carrot
- ¼ red pepper
- cilantro
- ½ tsp cinnamon
- 2 cups couscous
- 1 tsp olive oil

DIRECTIONS

1. Bring water boil add cumin, honey, cinnamon, add couscous and lemon juice

2. Cover and remove from heat
3. Add hers, olive oil, vegetables and serve

TOFU STICKS

Serves: *4*

Prep Time: *10* Minutes

Cook Time: *25* Minutes

Total Time: *35* Minutes

INGREDIENTS

- 1 tsp tamari sauce
- 1 tsp seasoning
- 1 cup tofu
- 1 tablespoon water
- ¼ cup cornflake crumbs

DIRECTIONS

1. In a bowl mix tamari with water
2. In another bowl mix cornflake and seasoning
3. Dip tofu into tamari sauce and then into seasoning
4. Place tofu slices on a baking sheet and bake at 325 for 15-18 minutes, remove and serve

BAKED EGGPLANT FRIES

Serves: **4**

Prep Time: **10** Minutes

Cook Time: **25** Minutes

Total Time: **35** Minutes

INGREDIENTS
- 1 eggplant
- 1 cup cornmeal
- ¼ tsp oregano
- ¼ tsp garlic powder
- ¼ tsp paprika
- 1 tsp olive oil
- 1 egg

DIRECTIONS

1. **Preheat oven to 375 F**
2. **In a bowl mix garlic powder, cornmeal, oregano and paprika**
3. **In a bowl beat the egg**
4. **Dip the eggplant fries in the beaten eggs and transfer to the cornmeal mixture**

5. Place the eggplant fried on a baking sheet and bake for 20 minutes, remove and serve

PITA CHIPS

Serves: **4**

Prep Time: **10** Minutes

Cook Time: **10** Minutes

Total Time: **20** Minutes

INGREDIENTS

- 2 pita rounds
- 2 tablespoons olive oil
- chili powder

DIRECTIONS

1. Cut each pita into 8 wedges
2. Brush with olive oil and sprinkle with chili powder
3. Bake at 325 F for 12 minutes or until crisp
4. Remove and serve

ROASTED RED PEPPER DIP

Serves: **2**

Prep Time: **10** Minutes

Cook Time: **10** Minutes

Total Time: **20** Minutes

INGREDIENTS

- 1 cup roasted red peppers
- 1 tablespoon olive oil
- 1 tsp lemon juice
- 1 clove garlic
- 1 tsp cumin

DIRECTIONS

1. In a blender mix all ingredients and blend until smooth
2. Remove and serve with pita chips

CHICKEN IN MUSHROOM SAUCE

Serves: **4**

Prep Time: **10** Minutes

Cook Time: **20** Minutes

Total Time: **30** Minutes

INGREDIENTS

- ½ cup all-purpose flour
- 1 tablespoon no-salt margarine
- 1 cup mushrooms
- 2 green onions
- pepper
- 1 tablespoon sour cream
- 1 tablespoon mustard
- 1 cup chicken broth
- 3 chicken breasts
- ½ dried thyme

DIRECTIONS

1. In a bowl mix chicken broth, flour, mustard, sour cream and set aside
2. Sprinkle with pepper, thyme and dredge in flour

3. Melt margarine in a pan and cook chicken for 5-6 minutes per side, remove and set aside
4. In a skillet add mushrooms, chicken broth and boil for 3-4 minutes
5. Whisk in sour cream mixture and onions
6. Pour mixture over chicken garnish with parsley and serve

BARBECUE CHICKEN SALAD

Serves: **2**

Prep Time: **10** Minutes

Cook Time: **50** Minutes

Total Time: **60** Minutes

INGREDIENTS

- 3 chicken breasts
- 1 tsp soy sauce
- 1 tablespoon olive oil
- 1 tablespoon cilantro
- 1 clove garlic
- ¼ tsp red chili pepper
- 2 yellow peppers
- 2 tablespoons rice vinegar
- 4 cups salad greens
- 1 tablespoon ginger

DIRECTIONS

1. In a bowl whisk soy sauce, cilantro pepper flakes, garlic and cilantro

2. Add chicken breasts and toss to coat, refrigerate for 30-45 minutes
3. Grill peppers for 12-15 minutes, remove to a plate
4. Place chicken breasts on grill and grill for 12-15 minutes per side on medium heat
5. Chop grilled peppers and chicken and place in salad bowl
6. Toss chicken, greens and peppers and serve

TUNA SPREAD

Serves: **2**

Prep Time: **10** Minutes

Cook Time: **10** Minutes

Total Time: **20** Minutes

INGREDIENTS

- 1 can no salt tuna
- 1 tablespoon mayonnaise
- 1 tsp lemon juice
- ¼ mustard
- pepper

DIRECTIONS

1. In a bowl mix all ingredients and season with pepper
2. When ready serve with toast

THAI SALAD

Serves: 2
Prep Time: 10 Minutes
Cook Time: 10 Minutes
Total Time: 20 Minutes

INGREDIENTS

- 1 tablespoon cornstarch
- 1 tablespoon ginger root
- 1 clove garlic
- 1 tsp sesame oil
- 1 lb. beef strip loin

SALAD

- 6 cups romaine lettuce
- 3 tsp canola oil
- ¼ cup grape tomatoes
- ½ cup cucumber

DIRECTIONS

1. In a bow mix ginger root, lime juice, garlic, cornstarch, sesame oil and chili sauce
2. Add beef and toss to coat

3. In another bowl mix salad ingredients
4. Pour over dressing and serve

PARSLEY PILAF

Serves: *4*

Prep Time: *10* Minutes

Cook Time: *20* Minutes

Total Time: *30* Minutes

INGREDIENTS

- 1 cup rice
- 1 tablespoon no-salt margarine
- 1 onion
- 1 cup chicken broth
- 1 tablespoon parsley

DIRECTIONS

1. In a pot add margarine, rice and onion, cook until golden brown
2. Add chicken broth and bring to boil
3. Reduce heat and cover, simmer until tender
4. Remove from heat, add parsley and serve

STEAMED FISH

Serves: **4**

Prep Time: **10** Minutes

Cook Time: **15** Minutes

Total Time: **25** Minutes

INGREDIENTS

- 3 fillets tilapia
- 1 tablespoon ketchup
- juice of half lemon
- 1 cup water
- ½ cup olive oil
- 2/4 cup green peppers
- ½ cup onion
- ½ tsp black pepper
- 1 tsp hot pepper sauce
- 1 spring thyme

DIRECTIONS

1. In a pan heat oil and sauté bell peppers and onion
2. Add thyme, ketchup, pepper, black pepper, lime juice and hot water and stir

3. Place fish in a pan and spoon vegetables
4. Cook for 10-12 minutes, remove and serve

SHRIMP STIR FRY

Serves: **4**

Prep Time: **10** Minutes

Cook Time: **30** Minutes

Total Time: **40** Minutes

INGREDIENTS

- ½ lb. shrimp
- ¾ Apple
- 2 celery stalks
- ¼ sweet red pepper
- 1 tablespoons vegetable oil

MARINADE

- ¼ tsp low sodium soy sauce
- 1 tsp cornstarch

SAUCE

- ¼ tsp low sodium soy sauce
- 1 tsp sugar
- 1 tsp cornstarch
- 1 tablespoon water

DIRECTIONS

1. Marinade the shrimp into the marinade ingredients
2. In a bowl mix sauce ingredients and set aside
3. In a wok fry shrimp, remove and set aside
4. In the same wok fry celery, red pepper and diced apple
5. Add in the shrimp, sauce mixture and stir until the sauce thickens
6. Remove and serve

DINNER

LOW POTASSIUM FRIED POTATOES

Serves: **2**

Prep Time: **10** Minutes

Cook Time: **15** Minutes

Total Time: **25** Minutes

INGREDIENTS

- 2 potatoes
- ¼ cup canola oil
- ¼ tsp paprika
- ¼ tsp white pepper
- 6 tsp ketchup

DIRECTIONS

1. Cut potatoes into small pieces
2. Heat oil in a skillet and add potatoes and cook for 8-10 minutes or until golden brown
3. Remove potatoes to a towel and set aside
4. In a bow mix paprika, white pepper and cumin
5. Sprinkle mixture over potatoes, toss and serve

STEWED POTATOES

Serves: **4**

Prep Time: **10** Minutes

Cook Time: **30** Minutes

Total Time: **40** Minutes

INGREDIENTS

- 2 cups potatoes
- ¼ tsp black pepper
- 1 tablespoon no-salt margarine
- 1 tsp white flour
- ¼ cup water
- ¼ cup nondairy creamer
- ½ tsp garlic powder

DIRECTIONS

1. Dice potatoes into small cubes and soak to reduce potassium
2. Place potatoes in a saucepan with water and boil for 12-15 minutes
3. Drain potatoes and return to pan, add nondairy creamer, onion powder, garlic, margarine, pepper and boil

4. Mix flour with water and stir into potatoes
5. Stir until liquid thickens, serve when ready

LOW POTASSIUM STIR-FRY

Serves: 2

Prep Time: 10 Minutes

Cook Time: 20 Minutes

Total Time: 30 Minutes

INGREDIENTS

- 3 cups mixed greens
- 6 oz. tofu
- ¼ tsp sesame oil
- ¼ tsp sesame seeds
- 1 tablespoon olive oil
- 1 cup onion
- ½ tsp curry powder
- 1 tsp soy sauce
- ¼ cup rice vinegar

DIRECTIONS

1. Cut greens into 1-inch shreds
2. In a wok heat oil, sauce onions for 2-3 minutes
3. Sprinkle curry powder over onions and add greens and sugar

4. Reduce heat and let greens steam until tender
5. Remove greens, add soy sauce, vinegar
6. Remove from heat, garnish with sesame oil and serve

LOW POTASSIUM SOY SAUCE

Serves: **2**

Prep Time: **10** Minutes

Cook Time: **10** Minutes

Total Time: **20** Minutes

INGREDIENTS

- 4 packets low sodium Boullion
- 5 tablespoons balsamic vinegar
- 4 tablespoons molasses
- 2 cups water
- ½ tsp black pepper
- ½ tsp powdered ginger
- ½ tsp garlic powder

DIRECTIONS

1. In a bowl mix all ingredients
2. Pour into a jar and refrigerate

GUACAMOLE

Serves: **2**

Prep Time: **10** Minutes

Cook Time: **10** Minutes

Total Time: **20** Minutes

INGREDIENTS

- 1 avocado
- 1 tablespoon lemon juice
- 1 tablespoon sour cream
- 1 tomato
- 1 onion
- ¼ tsp chili powder

DIRECTIONS

1. Mash avocado and mix with lemon juice
2. Add sour cream, onion, chili powder, tomato and stir
3. Chill and serve

GREEN PEA CASSEROLE

Serves: **4**

Prep Time: **10** Minutes

Cook Time: **30** Minutes

Total Time: **40** Minutes

INGREDIENTS

- 1 15 oz. can baby peas
- ½ cup onion
- ½ cup shredded cheddar cheese
- 1 cup crackers
- ¼ cup no-salt margarine
- 1 bottle dice pimento peppers
- 1 can sliced water chestnuts
- 1 can condensed cream of celery soup

DIRECTIONS

1. Preheat oven to 350 F
2. In a bowl mix water chestnut, peas, celery soup and onion
3. Pour into a casserole dish
4. Top with shredded cheese

5. In another bowl mix cracker and margarine, sprinkle over cheese
6. Bake for 30 minutes, remove and serve

TUNA CASSEROLE

Serves: 2

Prep Time: 10 Minutes

Cook Time: 30 Minutes

Total Time: 40 Minutes

INGREDIENTS

- 2 cups macaroni
- 1 can tuna
- 1 can condensed cream of chicken soup
- 1 cup cheddar cheese
- 1 cup fried onions

DIRECTIONS

1. Preheat oven to 325 F
2. In a baking dish mix soup, macaroni and tuna, top with cheese
3. Bake at 325 for 20-25 minutes
4. Sprinkle with onions and bake for another 2-3 minutes

PASTA SALAD

Serves: **2**

Prep Time: **10** Minutes

Cook Time: **10** Minutes

Total Time: **20** Minutes

INGREDIENTS

- 1 package pasta
- 1 cup salad dressing
- 1 cup parmesan cheese
- 1 red bell pepper
- 1 green bell pepper
- 1 onion

DIRECTIONS

1. In a pot cook pasta until al dente
2. In another bowl mix Italian salad dressing, pasta, salad dressing, parmesan cheese, green pepper, onion and red bell pepper
3. Mix well and serve

LINGUINE

Serves: 2

Prep Time: 10 Minutes

Cook Time: 20 Minutes

Total Time: 30 Minutes

INGREDIENTS

- 1 package linguine pasta
- 1 tablespoon olive oil
- ¾ cup butter
- 2 cloves garlic
- 1 tablespoon thyme leaves
- 4 roasted red peppers

DIRECTIONS

1. In a pot add linguine, olive oil, water and boil for 8-10 minutes until al dente
2. Melt butter in a saucepan, add garlic and cool until golden brown
3. Add thyme, red peppers, butter and cook for a couple of minutes
4. Pour over pasta and serve

SPAGHETTI WITH GARLIC

Serves: **2**

Prep Time: **10** Minutes

Cook Time: **20** Minutes

Total Time: **30** Minutes

INGREDIENTS

- 1 package spaghetti
- ½ cup olive oil
- ½ cup unsalted butter
- 3 cloves garlic
- 1 cup basil
- ½ cup parmesan cheese

DIRECTIONS

1. In a pot add spaghetti, water and cook for 10 minute until al dente
2. In another bowl toss spaghetti with butter, garlic, olive oil, basil and pepper
3. Serve with parmesan cheese

PIZZA

Serves: *4*

Prep Time: *10* Minutes

Cook Time: *30* Minutes

Total Time: *40* Minutes

INGREDIENTS

- 1 can pizza crust dough
- 1 tsp dill weed
- 1 tablespoon olive oil
- 4 mushrooms
- 1 cup sour cream
- 1 clove garlic
- 1 bell pepper
- ¾ cup baby spinach
- 1 cup cream cheese
- 1 onion

DIRECTIONS

1. **Preheat oven to 350 F**
2. **Place pizza dough on a baking sheet**

3. In a bowl mix cream cheese, sour cream and dill until smooth
4. Spread mixture over crust
5. In a skillet add mushrooms, onion, red bell pepper, garlic and stir for 4-5 minutes, stir in baby spinach
6. Spread mixture over the top of the pizza
7. Bake for 15-18 minutes or until golden brown
8. Remove and serve

RICE WITH HERBES

Serves: *4*

Prep Time: *10* Minutes

Cook Time: *20* Minutes

Total Time: *30* Minutes

INGREDIENTS

- 1 cup rice
- 1 cup chicken stock
- 1 tsp herbes de Provence
- 1 pinch pepper

DIRECTIONS

1. In a saucepan stir chicken stock, herbs, pepper and rice
2. Simmer over medium heat for 18-20 minutes
3. Remove and serve

BUFFALO CHICKEN DIP

Serves: **4**

Prep Time: **10** Minutes

Cook Time: **30** Minutes

Total Time: **40** Minutes

INGREDIENTS

- 2 cans chicken
- 2 packages cream cheese
- 1 cup dressing
- ¾ cup pepper sauce
- 1 cup cheddar cheese
- 1 bunch celery
- 1 box crackers

DIRECTIONS

1. In a skillet add chicken and sauce over medium heat
2. Stir in cream cheese and dressing
3. Add shredded cheese and transfer to a slow cooker
4. Cook on low for 6-8 hours or until done
5. Remove and serve with crackers

SAUTEED APPLES

Serves: *4*
Prep Time: *10* Minutes
Cook Time: *15* Minutes
Total Time: *25* Minutes

INGREDIENTS

- ½ cup butter
- ¼ cup water
- ¼ cup brown sugar
- ¼ tsp cinnamon
- 3 tart apples
- 1 tsp cornstarch

DIRECTIONS

1. In a skillet melt butter over medium heat
2. Add apples and cook until tender
3. Add cornstarch, stir in brown sugar and cinnamon
4. Boil for 2-3 minutes, remove and serve

CELERY STUFFING

Serves: **4**

Prep Time: **10** Minutes

Cook Time: **35** Minutes

Total Time: **45** Minutes

INGREDIENTS

- 1 lb. white bread
- 2 tsp poultry seasoning
- pepper
- 1 cup chicken broth
- ¾ cup unsalted butter
- 1 onion
- 3 stalks celery

DIRECTIONS

1. Cut bread slices into cubes
2. In a Dutch oven melt butter, add onion and celery
3. Season with poultry seasoning, pepper and stir in bread cubes
4. Bake in a casserole dish at 325 F for 35 minutes
5. Remove and serve

STUFFED JALAPENOS

Serves: 3
Prep Time: 10 Minutes
Cook Time: 25 Minutes
Total Time: 35 Minutes

INGREDIENTS

- 1 lb. pork sausage
- 1 package cream cheese
- 1 cup parmesan cheese
- 1 lb. jalapeno peppers
- 8 oz. ranch dressing

DIRECTIONS

1. Preheat oven to 400 F
2. In a skillet place sausage over medium heat
3. In a bowl mix cream cheese, parmesan cheese and sausage, spoon 1 tablespoon of mixture into jalapeno and place on a baking dish
4. Bake for 20-25 minutes
5. Remove and serve with dressing

FRIED CABBAGE

Serves: **3**

Prep Time: **10** Minutes

Cook Time: **15** Minutes

Total Time: **25** Minutes

INGREDIENTS

- 2 slices bacon
- ½ cup onion
- 5 cup cabbage
- 1 tablespoon water
- 1 pinch sugar
- pepper
- 1 tablespoon vinegar

DIRECTIONS

1. In a skillet add bacon, cook on medium heat and set aside
2. Add onion, cabbage and stir in pepper and sugar
3. Cook for 12-15 minutes
4. Remove and serve

ZUCCHINI BREAD

Serves: **6**

Prep Time: **10** Minutes

Cook Time: **50** Minutes

Total Time: **60** Minutes

INGREDIENTS

- 2 cups all-purpose flour
- 1 tsp baking soda
- 1 tsp baking powder
- 1 tablespoon cinnamon
- 2 eggs
- 1 cup vegetable oil
- 2 cups sugar
- 2 tsp vanilla extract
- 2 cups zucchini
- 1 cup walnuts

DIRECTIONS

1. **Preheat oven to 300 F**
2. **In a bowl mix cinnamon, baking powder, salt, soda and flour**

3. In another bowl beat eggs, sugar, vanilla and oil
4. Add to the creamed mixture and stir in zucchini and nuts
5. Pour batter into pans and bake for 40-50 minutes
6. Remove, cut into slices and serve

PINWHEELS

Serves: **4**

Prep Time: **10** Minutes

Cook Time: **10** Minutes

Total Time: **20** Minutes

INGREDIENTS

- 2 packages cream cheese
- 1 package ranch dressing mix
- 1 green onion
- 3 flour tortillas
- ¼ cup red bell pepper
- ¼ cup celery
- 1 can black olives
- ¼ cup cheddar cheese

DIRECTIONS

1. In a bowl mix green onion, ranch dressing and cream cheese
2. Spread mixture on each tortilla
3. Sprinkle celery, olives, cheese and celery
4. Wrap tortillas in aluminum foil

5. Chill overnight, slice the chilled rolls and serve

RICE PILAF

Serves: *4*

Prep Time: *10* Minutes

Cook Time: *30* Minutes

Total Time: *40* Minutes

INGREDIENTS

- 2 tablespoons butter
- ¼ cup pasta
- ¼ onion
- 1 clove garlic
- ¼ cup white rice
- 1 cup chicken broth

DIRECTIONS

1. In a skillet melt butter over medium heat, add pasta, onion, garlic and cook until becomes translucent
2. Mix in chicken broth and rice
3. Reduce heat and simmer until rice is tender
4. Remove from heat and serve

SNACKS & DRINKS

RASPBERRY PEAR SORBET

Serves: **4**

Prep Time: **10** Minutes

Cook Time: **30** Minutes

Total Time: **40** Minutes

INGREDIENTS

- ½ cup sugar
- 1 tablespoon pear
- fresh raspberries
- 1 pint raspberries
- 1 pear
- ½ cup lime juice

DIRECTIONS

1. In a saucepan bring water to boil and add sugar, simmer for 4-5 minutes, remove from heat and refrigerate
2. Puree pear, raspberries and lime juice, stir in syrup

3. Spread mixture into a baking pan and freeze for a couple of hours
4. Transfer to a container and freeze overnight
5. Serve with raspberries

RASPBERRY LIMEADE

Serves: 5
Prep Time: 5 Minutes
Cook Time: 5 Minutes
Total Time: 10 Minutes

INGREDIENTS

- 1 cup frozen raspberries
- 1 cup water
- ½ cup sugar
- 6 mint springs
- 1 cup lime juice
- 2 cups soda water

DIRECTIONS

1. **In a blender place all ingredients and blend until smooth**
2. **Pour smoothie in a glass and serve**

GRILLED CORN

Serves: 2
Prep Time: 10 Minutes
Cook Time: 15 Minutes
Total Time: 25 Minutes

INGREDIENTS

- ½ cup unsalted butter
- 1 tablespoon parsley
- 1 tablespoon chives
- 1 tsp dried thyme
- ¼ tsp cayenne pepper
- 6 ear sweet corn

DIRECTIONS

1. In a bowl mix all ingredients without corn
2. Spread mixture over each ear of corn
3. Grill for 10-12 minutes on medium heat
4. Remove and serve

CANDY GRAPES

Serves: **4**

Prep Time: **10** Minutes

Cook Time: **10** Minutes

Total Time: **20** Minutes

INGREDIENTS

- 1 box gelatin
- 1 cup water
- lemon juice

DIRECTIONS

1. **Place gelatin into a bowl**
2. **Dip a toothpick in water and roll in mix**
3. **Place in fridge to chill**
4. **Remove and serve**

GINGER COOKIES

Serves: *4*

Prep Time: *10* Minutes

Cook Time: *20* Minutes

Total Time: *30* Minutes

INGREDIENTS

- 2 cups white flour
- 1 tsp ginger
- 1 tsp baking soda
- 2/4 tsp cinnamon
- ¼ tsp cloves
- 2/3 cup butter
- 1 cup granulated sugar
- 2 egg whites
- 1/2cup honey

DIRECTIONS

1. Preheat oven to 325 F
2. In a bowl mix cloves, flour, cinnamon, ginger and baking soda

3. In another bowl mix butter with a mixer and beat 1 cup sugar
4. Add honey, egg whites, and stir flour mixture into egg mixture
5. Shape into balls and roll balls into sugar
6. Place them on a cookie sheet and bake for 10-12 minutes, remove and serve

PUMPKIN PIE

Serves: **4**

Prep Time: **10** Minutes

Cook Time: **60** Minutes

Total Time: **70** Minutes

INGREDIENTS

- Pumpkin pie filling
- 2 cups spaghetti squash
- ½ cup maple syrup
- ½ cup sugar
- ½ cup almond milk
- 1 tablespoon olive oil
- 2 tablespoon cornstarch
- 1 tsp pumpkin pie spice

DIRECTIONS

1. Preheat oven to 325 F and prepare pie filling
2. Add all pie ingredients in a blender and blend until smooth
3. Pour filling into pie crust and bake for 55-60 minutes
4. Remove from oven and let it chill before serving

APPLE CAKE

Serves: **6**

Prep Time: **10** Minutes

Cook Time: **50** Minutes

Total Time: **60** Minutes

INGREDIENTS

- 2 apples
- 2 tablespoons sugar
- cinnamon
- 2 eggs
- ½ cup sugar
- 2 tablespoons oil
- 1 tablespoon potato starch

DIRECTIONS

1. Slice apples and arrange then in a baking dish
2. Sprinkle with sugar and cinnamon
3. Beat eggs and sugar together
4. Add oil, potato starch, salt and mix well
5. Pour batter over apple slices

6. Bake for 325 F for 50-60 minutes
7. Remove and serve

CHOCOLATE CAKE

Serves: **4**

Prep Time: **10** Minutes

Cook Time: **30** Minutes

Total Time: **40** Minutes

INGREDIENTS

- 1 chocolate cake mix
- 1 box instant pudding mix
- 3 eggs
- ¼ cup canola oil
- ¼ cup warm water
- 1 cup cream
- 1 cup chocolate chips

DIRECTIONS

1. **Preheat oven to 325 F, and grease a pan**
2. **In a bowl place all ingredients and use a mixer on medium speed for 3-4 minutes or until all ingredients are fully incorporate into mixture**
3. **Pour mixture into pan**
4. **Bake for 50 minutes**

5. Remove and dust with powdered sugar before serving

BLUEBERRY SMOOTHIE

Serves: *1*
Prep Time: *5* Minutes
Cook Time: *5* Minutes
Total Time: *10* Minutes

INGREDIENTS

- ½ cup blueberries
- 1 cup milk
- 1 tsp honey
- 1 fresh mint
- ice cubes

DIRECTIONS

1. In a blender place all ingredients and blend until smooth
2. Pour smoothie in a glass and serve

PINEAPPLE SMOOTHIE

Serves: **1**

Prep Time: **5** Minutes

Cook Time: **5** Minutes

Total Time: **10** Minutes

INGREDIENTS

- ¾ cup pineapple
- 1 scoop vanilla protein powder
- ¼ cup water
- ice cubes

DIRECTIONS

1. In a blender place all ingredients and blend until smooth
2. Pour smoothie in a glass and serve

FRUITS SMOOTHIE

Serves: *1*

Prep Time: *5* Minutes

Cook Time: *5* Minutes

Total Time: *10* Minutes

INGREDIENTS

- 6 oz. caned fruit cocktail
- 2 scoops vanilla protein powder
- ½ cup water
- ice cubes

DIRECTIONS

1. **In a blender place all ingredients and blend until smooth**
2. **Pour smoothie in a glass and serve**

MIXED BERRY SMOOTHIE

Serves: **1**

Prep Time: **5** Minutes

Cook Time: **5** Minutes

Total Time: **10** Minutes

INGREDIENTS

- 3 oz. water
- 1 cup mixed berries
- ice cubes
- 1 cup cream topping

DIRECTIONS

1. **In a blender place all ingredients and blend until smooth**
2. **Pour smoothie in a glass and serve**

PEACH SMOOTHIE

Serves: *1*

Prep Time: *5* Minutes

Cook Time: *5* Minutes

Total Time: *10* Minutes

INGREDIENTS

- ½ cup ice
- 2 tablespoons powdered egg whites
- 2/4 cup peaches
- 1 tablespoon sugar

DIRECTIONS

1. **In a blender place all ingredients and blend until smooth**
2. **Pour smoothie in a glass and serve**

STRAWBERRY SMOOTHIE

Serves: *1*

Prep Time: *5* Minutes

Cook Time: *5* Minutes

Total Time: *10* Minutes

INGREDIENTS

- ¾ cup strawberries
- ½ cup egg whites
- ice cubes
- 1 tablespoon sugar

DIRECTIONS

1. **In a blender place all ingredients and blend until smooth**
2. **Pour smoothie in a glass and serve**

BANANA SMOOTHIE

Serves: *1*

Prep Time: *5* Minutes

Cook Time: *5* Minutes

Total Time: *10* Minutes

INGREDIENTS

- 1 banana
- ½ cup plain yogurt
- 1 cup milk
- 1 tablespoon honey
- 1 tablespoon oat

DIRECTIONS

1. **In a blender place all ingredients and blend until smooth**
2. **Pour smoothie in a glass and serve**

APPLE SMOOTHIE

Serves: *1*

Prep Time: *5* Minutes

Cook Time: *5* Minutes

Total Time: *10* Minutes

INGREDIENTS

- 1 apple
- 1 cup applesauce
- ½ cup plain yogurt
- 1 cup milk
- 1 tablespoon honey
- 1 tablespoon oat

DIRECTIONS

1. **In a blender place all ingredients and blend until smooth**
2. **Pour smoothie in a glass and serve**

EGG SHAKE

Serves: **1**

Prep Time: **5** Minutes

Cook Time: **5** Minutes

Total Time: **10** Minutes

INGREDIENTS

- ½ cup liquid egg product
- 1 cup non-diary whipped topping
- almond extract
- vanilla extract
- ¼ cup berries
- 1 banana

DIRECTIONS

1. **In a blender place all ingredients and blend until smooth**
2. **Pour smoothie in a glass and serve**

MANGO SMOOTHIE

Serves: **1**

Prep Time: **5** Minutes

Cook Time: **5** Minutes

Total Time: **10** Minutes

INGREDIENTS

- 1 mango
- ½ cup plain yogurt
- 1 cup milk
- 1 tablespoon honey
- 1 tablespoon oat

DIRECTIONS

1. **In a blender place all ingredients and blend until smooth**
2. **Pour smoothie in a glass and serve**